GENETIC FUTURES AND OUR SEARCH FOR WISDOM

Celia Deane-Drummond

Professor of Theology and the Biological Sciences

An Inaugural Lecture
Delivered at Chester College of Higher Education
on 27 November 2001

Chester Academic Press

First published 2007
by Chester Academic Press
Corporate Communications
University of Chester
Parkgate Road
Chester CH1 4BJ

Printed and bound in the UK by the
Learning Resources Print Unit,
University of Chester
Cover designed by the
Learning Resources Graphics Team
University of Chester

©Celia Deane-Drummont, 2007

All Rights Reserved
No part of this publication may be reproduced, stored in a
retrieval system or transmitted in any form or by any
means without the prior permission of the copyright
owner, other than as permitted by current UK legislation
or under the terms of a recognised copyright licensing
scheme

A catalogue record for this publication is available from
the British Library

GENETIC FUTURES AND OUR SEARCH FOR WISDOM

When the Principal asked me to name the title of the Chair I would like to receive, it only took a moment's thought for me to come up with the idea of "Theology and the Biological Sciences". If an inaugural lecture is supposed to be about summarising a lifetime's work in academia, then you are about to be disappointed. However, I will point briefly in this introduction to how I came to develop an interest in theology; in particular, how religious ideas are challenged by and serve to challenge the biological sciences. I realise now that even attempting the modest task of convincing those of you who are scientists that theology is in any way relevant to the study of science could itself be the subject of a lecture. On the other hand, theologians might feel sceptical about whether or not science really has anything to do with theology at all. After tracing a very short autobiography of my interest in this area, I will move into the discussion of a key area for current debate, namely genetics, ethics and theology. I hope to show by this example that there is room for dialogue. Moreover, dialogue is not only important; it is also necessary for both fields of study.

My academic career began as a research scientist, focusing particularly on the nitrogen nutrition of plants. I am not going to dwell on the details of the science; suffice it to say that work of this nature put me in the position of an interlocutor between ecologists and biotechnologists. One of the key biotechnologists who I met as a young scientist working on my doctorate was Dr, now Professor, Don Grierson, working in the research laboratories in the

School of Agriculture of Nottingham University, located in the remote village of Sutton Bonnington. This was one of the first centres in the UK to work actively to produce genetically modified tomatoes for commercial use. Grierson managed to modify the tomatoes so that they lacked an enzyme called polygalacturonase, which made them go soft following picking. You may have tasted Grierson's tomatoes, as Sainsbury's sold GM tomato paste between 1996 and 1999! After my doctorate, I moved to Vancouver to take up a postdoctoral position at the University, and I began serious study of theology at two centres based on the University's campus: namely, the Vancouver School of Theology and Regent College.

Once I moved back to England, I took up a post at Cambridge University and then at Durham University, but my interest in theology continued to grow and develop, though now I began to ask ethical questions about the nature of science. Why was there so much research concentrated on maximising growth of wheat and barley, when there were barley and wheat mountains? Why was the funding base shifting towards commercialisation and what impact was this having on the kinds of questions being asked by scientists? Certainly, at Durham University, there was a particular focus on plant genetics and research into the way bacteria can be used to transform the genetics of plant cells. Bacteria contain a single strand of circular deoxyribonucleic acid known as a plasmid. Plant scientists at Durham in the 1980s developed a technique for inserting particular genes into bacteria, and then infecting plant cells. Bacterial DNA incorporated into that of the host plant could be picked out using antibiotics, as only transformed plants carried the antibiotic resistant marker genes. On the surface, at least, this seemed to be a good idea: if ways could be found of making insecticides or other chemicals inside plants, then this should be more environmentally friendly than the use of commercial sprays. Unfortunately, life is never that simple, and the ecologists in the same department were worried that new genes could escape and alter the genetic composition of wild species, or even grow out of control. Their fears were not totally unfounded, since recent reports in the journal *Nature* have found that genetically transformed corn escaped into the wild in Mexico, as did unregulated transformed cotton in India. The issue becomes not just scientific, but also sociopolitical. E. A. Siddiq, chairman of an Indian department of biotechnology, gives a salutatory warning about the dangers in this case: "This is a foretaste of a frightening situation where transgenics will be out of control all over the place".[1]

Traditionally, scientists have tried to detach themselves from responsibility for what happens to their own creations. Science discovers what is there, but technology then applies the knowledge in ways dependent on social and economic forces. However, I suggest that it is inappropriate for scientists to detach themselves from all responsibility or to expect "society" simply to take up consideration of ethics at the point at which science leaves off. Scientists are not just scientists, they are also citizens. Of course, some scientists have speculated freely about the wider consequences of their science. James Watson and Francis Crick's discovery of the double helical structure of deoxyribonucleic acid in 1953 was a landmark in the history of genetics. Soon afterwards, genetic scientists began to speculate about the possibility for the future genetic transformation of the *human race*. Scientists then were worried about what they saw as the potential disaster facing humanity, as the ability of medicine to keep those with genetic defects alive would in effect increase the

---

[1] E.A. Siddiq (as cited in *Nature*, 413 [11 October 2001], 555).

deleterious genetic load on human evolution. In the late 1950s, the American geneticist H. J. Muller predicted a future genetic apocalypse: "... the then existing germ cells of what were once human beings would be a lot of hopeless, utterly diverse genetic monstrosities".[2]

How might we tackle such a problem? Two possibilities exist:

- Genetic surgery of deleterious genes or insertion of desirable genes through "germ line" therapy;
- Preventative measures through social change; i.e., parental choice.

Greater awareness of the spectre of eugenics of the kind practiced in the Nazi era has made most geneticists wary of any enforced political implementation of genetic control of humans. Hence, even Muller is insistent that genetic change should be achieved through *voluntary* means, rather than coercion.

Textbooks in human genetic science today are likely to be far more cautious about making *any* social recommendations for the human race. Even the idea of preventative measures through social change does not square well with contemporary understanding of population genetics: "... the simplest equations of population genetics show that preventing people with rare recessive disorders from reproducing will *not* significantly reduce the frequency of these detrimental genes". [3]

If we ask the question, "What are the possibilities for genetic science?" to contemporary geneticists, the reply is more often than not that human genetics, at least, is

---

[2] H. J. Muller, 'The Guidance of Human Evolution', *Perspectives in Biology and Medicine*, 3 (1959), 1-43 (p. 11).
[3] Arthur P. Mange and Elaine Johansen Mange, *Genetics: Human Aspects*, 2nd edn (Sunderland, MA: Sinauer Associates, 1990), p. 10.

significant for medical science, rather than for any grand plan for eugenics. By focusing on particular instances of genetic disease, the possibility of medical treatment of severe conditions such as cystic fibrosis or Huntington's disease comes closer to reality. Even the susceptibility to more general diseases, such as some cancers, various forms of heart disease and a host of other medical conditions, has a genetic component. The idea that genetic science could alleviate an individual's suffering is one that has particular appeal. The geneticist Duncan Shaw suggests: "... we can look forward to a new era in molecular medicine, where intervention at the level of the gene will provide new opportunities for conquering some of the most intractable conditions known to medicine".[4]

The Human Genome Project boosted this optimism further. The HGP is a multimillion-dollar project carried out at an international level, with the intention of mapping the genetic sequence of the entire human genome. It was finished in a rough draft form in June 2000, though a more complete version was published earlier this year.[5] Optimism in the possibilities for genetics abound. More importantly, as far as geneticists are concerned, we would be irresponsible not to use genetics to improve the human condition. For:

> Until now we had no control over this random distribution. The genetic material we have been awarded is the result of a lottery, the lottery of life. Today we have the power to manipulate the genetic

---

[4] *Molecular Genetics of Human Inherited Disease*, ed. by Duncan J. Shaw (Chichester: John Wiley, 1995), p. 4.
[5] i.e., 2001.

material at will, to modify what it took Nature 4.5 billion years to create. These are exciting, but scary times.[6]

James Watson, co-discoverer of the structure of DNA, is one of the most outspoken geneticists in support of the prospect of using genetic technology to alter human genetics. The moral consequences of *not* using the knowledge are, for him, just as significant as focusing on the possible risks and dangers. Common diseases such as arteriosclerosis, Alzheimer's disease, diabetes and many cancers all have a genetic component. That is, a person's genes predispose them to a disease, along with unfavourable environmental factors, including diet.

Watson recognised that there are important social issues emerging from this new knowledge. For example: what use would be made of genetic propensity to disease by insurance companies or employers?; how would we come to terms with features of our own genetic lineage? While genetic tests might show a propensity to disease, for example, for many diseases there is little prospect of a cure. The allocation of first 3% and then 5% of funding to support the ethical, legal and social issues [ELSI] of the Human Genome Project was enough to show that such issues were being taken seriously, though small enough to ensure that the Project itself was not under threat.

There is still a legal barrier preventing geneticists from altering human germ cells; that is, eggs and sperm. Perhaps it is biology's last taboo. Watson believes that no government wants to take responsibility for initiating steps that serve to redirect human evolution. But for him, we should never put off doing something where risks are

---

[6] Philippe Frossard, *The Lottery of Life: The New Genetics and the Future of Mankind* (London: Bantam Press, 1991), p. 13.

unknown. He dismisses the idea that we are going to produce "super persons" but, at the same time:

> If appropriate go-ahead signals come, the first resulting gene-bettered children will in no sense threaten human civilization. They will be seen as special only in their immediate circles, and are likely to pass as unnoticed in later life as the now grownup "test-tube baby" Louise Brown does today....
>
> Moving forward will not be for the faint of heart. But if the next century witnesses failure, let it be because our science is not yet up to the job, not because we don't have the courage to make less random the sometimes most unfair courses of human evolution.[7]

Is such enthusiasm justified? Cloning is a case in point. While most reject the idea of human reproductive cloning, the use of cloned eggs for therapeutic medical purposes was recently approved in the UK. The 14 day cut-off period relates to the appearance of the primitive streak in the embryo, which some scientists prefer to call an "ovasome", as it is derived though nuclear transfer rather than fertilisation as such. However, the real possibility of the use of therapeutic cloning to treat human diseases is not now thought to have much clinical impact. The reason for this is that therapeutic cloning is unlikely to be commercially viable, relying as it does on the donation of eggs.[8] Therapeutic cloning depends on the production of totipotent cells, known as stem cells, which form early in

---

[7] James Watson, *A Passion for DNA: Genes, Genomes, and Society* (Oxford: Oxford University Press, 2000), p. 229.
[8] Peter Aldhous, 'Can They Rebuild Us?', *Nature*, 410 (5 April 2001), 622-625.

the development of a clone or embryo. However, more ethically acceptable ways of harvesting stem cells are currently being developed, either from mature tissues of the patient or from other tissues lines genetically engineered, so that they are not targeted by the body's natural immune system, without any need to create a "clone" first. While these stem cells are less effective than those derived from early embryos or "ovasomes", the practical and ethical difficulties in the latter case outweigh its scientific advantages. Much of this work is under a cloak of commercial secrecy. Private companies have started offering new mothers the opportunity to bank cord blood, also a source of stem cells, for possible future treatment of their child. The probability that such blood could be used is very small and many doctors are worried that this just plays on the natural vulnerability and fears of new mothers.

Perhaps Dolly, the first cloned sheep, is symbolic of the new genetics. It was through the efforts of a commercial company that the cloning of a mammal was achieved. However, the purpose of the cloning technique was to find a practical way out of a practical problem; namely, to find an efficient way of making genetically altered sheep, engineered with different human genes. In much the same way, cloning in humans is likely to be supported by geneticists, not so much as a way of reproducing identical individuals, but as a way forward in altering the germ line.[9] The most likely scenario is that a modified version of *in vitro* fertilisation will be used and single cells extracted to test for genetic change prior to implantation. Of course, manipulation of animal germ cells has been practised for some time; in this case, foreign DNA would be injected

---

[9] Jonathan Knight, 'Biology's Last Taboo', *Nature*, 413 (6 September 2001), 12-15.

directly into the egg cells. Some cells would be transformed and take up other genes, in this case those of a rat. It is a sobering fact that a large percentage of our DNA is remarkably similar to that of other species. Not only are we 98% similar to chimpanzees, but our proud species contains a paltry 30,000 genes, about twice that of the fruit fly. Even nematode worms share 60% of human genes.[10] However, it is very unlikely that similar techniques would be used with humans at the moment, because of the high risk of malformations. Even the use of such experimental methods in animals raises important issues of animal welfare.

What are the more specific ethical questions about the future possibilities in genetic science? I suggest that questions need to be asked now, before such technologies become routine and established and before there is general acceptance that change is permissible in the way that Watson indicated, for the possible control of the future course of human evolution through genetics is not just an issue for genetic science alone. I would like to pose some questions to James Watson. In the first place: should we necessarily just use the genetic calculus in making decisions about what ought to be done? In this case, the absolutely imperative end is that of genetic control or improvement. Certainly, if one has a passion for DNA and nothing else, as seems to be the case with James Watson, it might seem like a sensible way forward. But I suggest that there are other ways of considering our futures, which open up problems that cannot be quantified by a simple calculation of risk and benefit. Do we really want to be able to design our own children according to preset characteristics? While the initial focus of genetic science

---

[10] S. Franklin, 'Gene answer spawns a lot of questions', *The Times Higher Educational Supplement*, 15 June 2001, p. 19.

will, rightly in my view, be on the elimination of deleterious genes, how far does the desire to control our future represent a false hope; one that is bound to fail?

Certainly, Philippe Frossard, writing as one with experience in genetic science, argues that more humane goals in genetics are readily eclipsed by commercial interests. Therapeutic cloning is a case in point. He remarks:

> I have always had the uneasy feeling that the potential of a drug to treat human disease is a fortuitous side effect, a marketable commodity that helps win over media attention while the primary goal concerns two of the strongest motivating factors; greed and ambition.[11]

His comments were made before the Human Genome Project was completed. Yet, even in this case, the commercial rush to patent different parts of the human genome for profit was exploited by a certain individual. Craig Venter set up his own private company, called Celera Genomics, in order to complete the sequence ahead of the publicly funded programme. The ethical issue remains: how far are companies justified in patenting parts of the human genome? For example, the patent for one of the breast cancer genes, BRCA1, is held by a company called Myriad. This means that, in practice, laboratories screening for breast cancer genes should pay Myriad a fee. While those in the USA have complied, Europeans are generally defiant. Otmar Kloiber of the German Medical Association states: "The substance patents now being given to the human genome are inappropriate and endanger research and medicine. Information about the human

---

[11] Frossard, p. 225.

genome can't be invented. It is the common heritage of all humans".[12] The ethical questions about the use of genetic knowledge for good or ill are not, then, simply questions of assessing the real benefits as against unknown or unquantifiable risks. If we frame ethical questions in this way, then we are adopting a particular philosophical stance known as consequentialism. I suggest that when issues are presented in such a way, the presentation is loaded towards genetic change. Rather, I suggest that the *motivation* of those engaged in such tasks needs to be taken into account in any analysis of the likely scenarios portrayed by such visions.

Even James Watson presents the medical case for the Human Genome Project as that which is most likely to win over public support. The issue of whether or not to go ahead is not seriously challenged. Yet, even from within science, there are more cautious voices; for if it has taken 4.5 billion years for *Homo sapiens* to emerge, deliberately trying to alter the course of our evolution may have highly unpredictable effects. The earliest scientists were also those who took philosophy and theology seriously. The historian of science John Brooke reminds us that the portrayal of science as being in opposition to religious truth is historically inaccurate.[13] Nonetheless, the geneticists of today are more likely to be atheists. James Watson, like Richard Dawkins, wishes to exclude all religious and most other public considerations of genetics. I suggest that such a narrowing of vision amounts to a disservice to genetics, for a wider appreciation of the religious, ethical, social and political concerns about who we are, as persons, can begin to put our genetic discoveries in perspective. We are more

---

[12] Otmar Kloiber (as cited in *Nature*, 413 [4 October, 2001], 443).
[13] John Hedley Brooke, *Of Scientists and Their Gods: An Inaugural Lecture Delivered before the University of Oxford on 21 November, 2000* (Oxford: Oxford University Pres, 2001).

than just our genes. I suggest that genetic science needs to be qualified by an accompanying search, namely that of wisdom. Wisdom is that elusive quality that seeks to see everything in relation to everything else. This need not exclude scientific discoveries, but it puts scientific truth alongside other ways of knowing and thinking.

The philosopher Mary Midgley insists that at the heart of all knowledge there must be a sense of goodness, as this shows the point of all other knowledge.[14] Modern science, she suggests, has lost this contemplative stance; it is always straining ahead to the new, instead of reflecting on the significance of what is there already. Nicholas Lash, from Cambridge University, makes a similar point; namely, that our ingenuity has outstripped our wisdom.[15] Theology in the service of science is not just affirming what science is doing or will do, but reminding it to reconsider the place of its own knowledge in the context of other ways of knowing.

In seeking after theological resources for wisdom, I suggest that the medieval synthesis of Thomas Aquinas, who combined the philosophy of Aristotle, often thought to be the pioneer of modern biology, with that of the Early Church Father Saint Augustine of Hippo, offers promising insights that are relevant for today.[16] Of course, there are other ways of thinking about wisdom from a theological point of view, but they would be the subject of another lecture. For Aquinas, wisdom is one of the intellectual virtues. Reason is both speculative and practical. The three virtues of speculative reason are *wisdom, scientia* and

---

[14] Mary Midgley, *Wisdom, Information and Wonder; What is Knowledge For?* (London: Routledge, 1989), pp. 13-14.
[15] Nicholas Lash, *The Beginning and the End of "Religion"* (Cambridge: Cambridge University Press, 1996), pp. 116-117.
[16] Celia Deane-Drummond, *Creation Through Wisdom: Theology and the New Biology* (Edinburgh: T&T Clark, 2000).

understanding. *Scientia* is the comprehension of the causes of things and the relationship between them. *Understanding* means grasping first principles. *Wisdom* is the understanding of the fundamental causes of everything and their relationship to everything else. It informs both speculative and practical reason. The two virtues of practical reason are prudence and art. Practical wisdom or prudence is a clear perception of reality directed towards the good, leading to practical action. Art, on the other hand, is perfection in the art of judging.

For Aquinas, the fundamental cause is God, so wisdom is ultimately knowledge of God's nature and actions. In the end, then, the wisdom ethic that Aquinas develops is a theocentric one, even though he does not deny the use of human reason. I suggest that it is this appreciation of the use of reason, combined with an awareness of both practical issues and the intimacy of the presence of God, which makes the wisdom ethic particularly instructive in unravelling the dilemmas facing us in the new biology. For *scientia* alone will tend to draw us simply to a risk/benefit approach to ethics. In those cases in which the risks are unknown or unquantified, this slants action in favour of change.

On the other hand, when theological reflection simply condemns genetic science by making statements of principle, such as, "It is Wrong to Play God", this leads to the kind of hostility towards religion that is found in the likes of geneticists such as Richard Dawkins or James Watson. Statements of principle could quite easily be directed in support of genetic engineering, rather than against it. Francis Collins, who took over from James Watson as the head of the Human Genome Project in the USA, is rare amongst prominent geneticists in that he is also a committed Christian. He suggests that human genetic change is part of our Christian mandate to heal the sick, in imitation of Christ.[17] However, the more interesting question is how we come to make decisions when there are conflicting interests. For this, I suggest that we need to develop the art of practical wisdom, or prudence. What, then, is prudence? Aquinas believed that the true end of all the virtues is goodness and, loosely speaking, we can think of prudence as the means of attaining this end. Prudence is a clear perception of reality and is required for the practice of all the other moral virtues; namely, courage, justice and temperance. However, in many cases we cannot separate the goal of a virtue from the action or practice of it. In other words, the means and the ends are closely intertwined. The task of prudence becomes what Aquinas describes as discerning through the use of reason the right course of action, in order to express a particular virtue, both for the good of the individual and the good of the community.

Keeping the balance between the good of the individual and of the community is particularly challenging when addressing issues in the new biology, as I have indicated earlier. It is important, too, to see prudence in alignment with justice, temperance and courage. Justice is of particular significance, for rational action without justice is not a real act of prudence. In considering the aims of genetic engineering, we need to ask ourselves how far this coheres with issues of justice between groups of people. What does the desire for genetic perfection say about how we value those who are not genetically perfect? Tom Shakespeare, of the Policy, Ethics and Life Sciences Institute at Newcastle University, suffers from a genetic disease known as achondroplasia. He argues that both he and his daughter have a quality of life

---

[17] F. S. Collins, 'The Human Genome Project: Tool of Atheistic Reductionism or Embodiment of the Christian Mandate to Heal?', *Science & Christian Belief*, 11 (1999), 99-112.

that Watson seems to assume cannot be theirs.[18] Watson, in claiming that "... terminating the existence of a genetically disabled fetus ... is incomparably more compassionate than allowing an infant to come into the world tragically impaired"[19], too readily lumps all genetic defects together and assumes that physical perfection is the goal of human existence. However, being genetically damaged in some way is virtually inevitable for every member of the human race. It is those qualities that we select for change that say something about our ability or otherwise to exercise prudence. How do we make prudential choices? Should we, as Watson assumes, positively introduce qualities into our children, such as enhanced intelligence? If this becomes the aim of genetic science, then courage is needed in challenging those aspects of the status quo that go against the aim of justice. The notion of temperance, although perhaps unpopular today, is an important quality to align with prudence, in that it implies self-restraint. It is far too easy to assume that the goods I pursue for my own ends are self-evident, without proper consideration of how this might affect others in the community, both in the human and the natural world. Wisdom is a reminder of this polyvalence in goodness; the fact that what might be "the good" for the individual must be balanced with "the good" for the community as a whole.

Another aspect of prudence that emerges in the thought of Aquinas is the ability to have a clear perception of reality in a specific situation. This requires virtues that Aquinas describes as allied to that of prudence: namely, memory of the past, insight into the present and shrewdness about the future, along with reason,

---

[18] T. Shakespeare, 'No Hope of Reality Modifying Brilliance', 19 January 2001, *The Times Higher Educational Supplement*, p. 27.
[19] Watson, p. 225.

understanding, openness to being taught, circumspection and caution. The idea of any precautionary principle seems to be anathema to influential scientists like James Watson. He considers in retrospect that a moratorium on recombinant DNA research in the early 1970s was a mistake; all that discussion did was to delay progress. However, this seems to be a very selective use of memory. The family of Jesse Gelsinger,[20] who died as a result of a somatic gene therapy experiment, would not agree with Watson's cavalier approach. Jesse Gelsinger suffered from a mild form of ornithine transcarbamylase deficiency, but volunteered to help in the interests of scientific research. For prudence, the need for memory of the past is both individual and collective, so that, if either of these memories is suppressed or obscured, insight into the present is impaired, along with a distorted assessment of goals for the future. Prudence gives us the habit that allows us to compare any new situations with old and, by noticing differences between them, it allows us to act appropriately for the good. It helps us notice very subtle differences in situations, rather than simply applying certain rules and generalisations from past experiences. Genetic changes that are advocated now are certainly not identical with those of Nazi Germany, but the memory of the failures of eugenics serves as a salutary warning about how not to proceed.

---

[20] Jesse Gilsinger suffered from a mild form of ornithine transcarbamylase deficiency. It is a disorder of nitrogen metabolism that could be controlled by drugs. Researchers used adenoviruses to transform his genes, and his death was a result of an immune response to viral vectors. None of the patients showed significant gene expression and only 1% reached target cells. It might have been foreseeable, as monkeys had died in trials and he was wrongly told it would be clinically beneficial. (See Julian Savulescu, 'Harm, Ethics Committees and the Gene Therapy Death: Editorial 2', *The Journal of Medical Ethics*, 27 [2001], 148-150.)

Prudence, or practical wisdom, encourages a flexibility in thought that is very different from the conditioned responses preprogrammed by past experience. I suggest that such subtlety is a much needed quality when facing complex issues in the new biology. While we are reminded constantly of the newness of the techniques that are now possible, a historical appreciation of the ways new science has become used or abused in the past may help us to find ways forward. This is not the same as nostalgia about the past, but a question of learning from past mistakes and past experiences. What is a wisdom ethic? Wisdom relies on the sum of the cultural learning of past generations; it is an expression of maturity that is prepared to be patient, rather than automatically welcoming all that is novel and different. However, at the same time, it reflects an attitude that is open to the possibility for the good. This means that a wisdom ethic will not automatically condemn genetic engineering out of hand, but consider it carefully in the light of past experiences and possibilities for the future.

Moreover, from the perspective of Christian theology, the new genetics challenges a re-visioning of who God is, wisdom being the fundamental characteristic of God's Being as well as God's Action. Just as wisdom is the means through which God creates the world, so any human desire for its re-creation needs to look to the fundamental Wisdom of God. What this wisdom is and how it might be expressed in terms of Christian theology would be the subject of another lecture. Suffice it to say that thinking about God in terms of wisdom engages both ancient Orthodox ideas, as well as those in medieval theology that I have alluded to here, alongside contemporary feminist understanding.[21] Yet I suggest that the search for wisdom is one that is inclusive of the whole community; it is *our*

---

[21] Deane-Drummond, *Creation Through Wisdom*.

search for wisdom, not theology's search or science's search. Public concern about genetic engineering in itself creates an implicit theology, one that it would be prudent for policy makers to take seriously.[22] Theology can serve to remind us of the difficulty of the task. In the words of Quoholeth: "Whatever wisdom may be, it is far off and most profound - who can discover it?" (Ecclesiastes 7.24).

---

[22] Celia Deane-Drummond, Robin Grove White and Bronislaw Szerszynski, 'Genetically Modified Theology: The Religious Dimensions of Public Concerns about Agricultural Biotechnology', *Studies in Christian Ethics*, 14 (2001), 23-41.